Moringa Over Medicine

"There is a Plant for Every Illness."

Dexter & Petula Jones

Moringa Over Medicine

Uwriteitpublishing Company
Goldsboro, NC 27534

Moringa Over Medication by Dexter & Petula Jones
Copyright © 2018 Dexter & Petula Jones

ALL RIGHTS RESERVED

ISBN-13: 978-1729538531

ISBN-10: 1729538533

First Printing—November 2018

NO PART OF THIS BOOK MAY BE REPRODUCED IN ANY FORM, BY PHOTOCOPYING OR BY ANY ELECTRONIC OR MECHANICAL MEANS, INCLUDING INFORMATION STORAGE OR RETREVIAL SYSTEMS, WITHOUT PERMISSION IN WRITING FROM THE COPYRIGHT OWNER/AUTHOR.

This publication is designed to provide information in regard to the subject matter covered. It is published with the understanding that the author is not engaged in rendering legal counsel or other professional services. It is for educational purposes only. If legal advice or other professional advice is required, the services of a professional person should be sought.

- These statements have not been evaluated by the Food & Drug Administration. This product information is not intended to diagnose, treat, cure or prevent any diseases.
- Scripture quotations are from the King James Version of the Bible unless otherwise stated.

Moringa Over Medicine

"Let Moringa be your medicine and your medicine be Moringa."

"America is sicker than ever because she has blindly turned her will over to medicine without reasoning if medicine is the best option."

Moringa Over Medicine

"He causeth the grass to grow for the cattle, and herb for the service (the aid, assistance and help) of man: that he may bring forth food out of the earth." Psalms 104:14

Moringa Over Medicine

"In 2018 Americans spent $360.2 Billion dollars so far on prescription drugs."

Moringa Over Medicine

"Moringa is the most powerful superfood ever discovered by mankind. It's the only plant that supplies our bodies with all the essential nutrients needed for a healthy body in one single plant."

Moringa Over Medicine

"It has been estimated that by 2021 spending will be between $400-$600 billion for prescription medicine according to a report released by Quintiles IMS. So things aren't getting better they're getting worse.

Moringa Over Medicine

"Moringa Oleifera is often called "The Miracle Tree" because of the enormous health benefits that one derives from using it."

Moringa Over Medicine

Table of Contents

Acknowledgements
About the Authors
First Partakers

1. Sickness in America
2. The Truth About Medicine
3. The Truth About Moringa Oleifera
4. Moringa Over Medicine
5. God's Spiritual Superfood
6. A New You Today, The Moringa Way
7. You Are Fearfully and Wonderfully Made

Acknowledgements

I would like to first off acknowledge the Creator and Maker of all plant life and human life—God Almighty. Whatever mankind thinks he has discovered he has only brought to the surface God's creation and therefore the honor and glory belongs to God Almighty. Moringa Oleifera is God's plant and we're privileged to be able to distribute and sell it to help individuals to meet their health and wellness needs and to get their health back. We acknowledge all our customers that has patronize our business in the past and that will patronize it in the future. God bless you all.

About the Authors

Dexter & Petula Jones is first and foremost Ministers of the gospel of Jesus Christ. Evangelists, that believes in going beyond the church walls to reach the lost with the good news of the gospel. Ministry is their first love because God saved them both out of a world of sin and transformed their lives and made them righteous through Jesus Christ. Now they're going about their Father's business letting the world know that Jesus is the Savior of the world and he came to reconcile man back to God.

Their second love is spreading the good news about God's Superfood Moringa Oleifera. This amazing product has changed their life physically and has enabled them to live a healthy life as well as a life of prevention from sickness and diseases. They know firsthand that the goal is wellness and prevention of disease rather than restoring health to a sick body.

The testimonies that they've seen from

Individuals that have used Moringa Oleifera on a consistent basis are in many instances amazing.

The manner in which God brought his creation into their hands is also amazing. In August of 2016 a friend of Dexter's nephew Jomo Jones whose name is Kelo was in town coming from Charlotte and he brought some Moringa back in town with him. He introduced all of us to the product and made us a bottle of Moringa water. He was very positive about the benefits of the product and what it had done for him and many other individuals whose testimonies he heard. So he gave us a bottle of Moringa water and after drinking it the product gave me instant energy. My response was, **"what is in this stuff?"** Kelo gave us each a sample to take home to continue to try it in order to reap all the benefits of this amazing plant.

As a God gifted researcher I begin to delve into the history of **"Moringa Oleifera"** and the more I researched the more amazed I became. Day by day I was learning new information about a product that I had never heard of before. I became obsessed with learning about this product that had changed the life of so many people. The more I learned the more I wanted to learn because I could not believe that one product could do all this. I have studied many herbs for 30 + years but nothing had even come close to Moringa Oleifera in a single plant.

Other herbs it was necessary in many instances to add many herbs together to get the full effect, Moringa Oliefera however was able to stand alone and yet supply the body with all the essential nutrients. This plant was truly amazing and the more I researched the deeper it got as I learned that over 1300 articles have been written about Moringa Oleifera as well as many books about the veracity of this superfood.

My ultimate conclusion was this is too good to keep to myself. I have to let the world (or at least my world and as my as I could reach) know about this plant that can do so many things but has been hidden for many years. I told my wife

Moringa Over Medicine

that this was more than just a great product that came into our hands, we have to get the word out. So after going through different processes of selling and distributing Moringa Oleifera we decided to make it a real business and formulate all the legalities we needed to establish our own health store called **"Eden Wellness Moringa."** We named it this because we believe that such a tree must have been in the **"Garden of Eden"** when God created his world and placed the man whom he formed. As the scripture states, *"And the LORD God formed man of the dust of the ground, and breathed into his nostrils the breath of life: and man became a living soul. And the LORD God planted a garden eastward in Eden; and there he put the man whom he had formed. And out of the ground made the LORD God to grow every tree **(the Moringa Tree)** that is pleasant to the sight, and good for food; the tree of life also in the midst of the garden, and the tree of the knowledge of good and evil. And a river went out of Eden to water the garden." Genesis 2:7-10a*

This was the beginning of both Ministry and Business for us to introduce Moringa Oleifera to the world.

FOREWORD

Moringa over Medicine is a book that will educate the reader about man's need to get back to the *"herb of the field." Genesis 3:18b* We have become a nation that is consumed with medicine and we're not the better for it. We're more doped up than ever before in spite of our advance in technology and the fact that mankind is smarter than ever.

Every medicine that comes on the market has a list of side effects that are sometimes worse off than the disease it's supposed to help. While the medicine is supposed to help one thing it can cause adverse defects in a number of other things. And the sad reality is that these side effects can range from:

1. Diarrhea
2. Headaches
3. Insomnia
4. Dizziness

Moringa Over Medicine

5. Drowsiness
6. Suicidal thoughts
7. Cancer
8. Nausea
9. And even Death, just to name a few.

These are medicines that are approved by the FDA for our taking with the understanding that if too many people have adverse side effects they will be taken off the market. Here are some cases in point that are just horrific when you think about it and the effects of them were astronomical. Let's look at the Medications that was approved and later taken off the market but left carnage of side effects and deaths in its tracks killing thousands of people.

1. *Baycol for cholesterol killed 52. (3 years on the market).*

2. *Propulsid for reflux disease killed 70.*

3. *Rezulin for Antidiabetic and anti-inflammatory killed 63.*

Moringa Over Medicine

4. *Selacryn killed 36 deaths; at least 500 cases of severe liver and kidney damage (3 years on the market).*

5. *Vioxx for pain relief killed about 60,000 and caused 140,000 heart attacks. (5.3 years on the market).*

6. *Darvon & Darvocet for Opioid pain reliever killed 2110. (55 years on the market).*

7. *Durat for pain killer 4 deaths; 8 patients requiring liver transplants; 12 patients with severe liver damage. (1 year on the market).*

8. *Lotronex for Irritable bowel syndrome (IBS) in women 49 cases of ischemic colitis (inflammation and injury of the large intestine); 21 cases of severe constipation (10 requiring surgery); 5 deaths; mesenteric ischemia (inflammation and injury of the small intestine) (8 months on the market).*

9. *Omniflox--Antibiotic for pneumonia, bronchitis, and other respiratory tract infections; prostatitis and other*

Moringa Over Medicine

genitourinary tract infections; skin ailments. This product caused 3 deaths; severe low blood sugar; hemolytic anemia and other blood cell abnormalities; kidney dysfunction (half of the cases required renal dialysis); allergic reactions including some causing life-threatening respiratory distress.

10. Propulsid--Severe nighttime heartburn associated with gastroesophageal reflux disease (GERD). This product caused more than 270 cases of serious cardiac arrythmias (including ventricular tachycardia, ventricular fibrillation, torsades de pointes, and QT prolongation) reported between July 1993 and May 1999, with 70 being deaths.

11. Moringa Oleifera--A natural plant that has been used for over 300 different sicknesses and diseases. Moringa Oleifera has been used for over 4000 years and has caused neither NO DEATHS nor any adverse side effects!

Moringa Over Medicine

What are we saying here? It's all about the money when it comes to medicine not necessarily about getting a cure for that sickness or disease. It seems as if daily, weekly, monthly and yearly they're coming out with new drugs that are supposed to be the answer for a certain sickness/disease. Only to find out years later that the adverse side effects did more harm than good. The reason I say more harm is because if 1 death is the result of side effects it's too many.

Well in this book we will bring forth the truth with the hopes that you will receive the truth and as the word of God states in revealing truth; *And ye shall know the truth, and the truth shall make you free."* *John 8:32* But just knowing truth without applying truth and making that truth a part of your life will keep your in error. The word of God wants you to not just know truth but become intimate with that truth and allow it to change your life. Our hope for you dear reader is the same, allow this truth to become applicable in your life and help create a new you.

"Seeing a sick body restored back to health is a good thing. However, what is better than restoration is a body that remains healthy consistently."

First Partakers

"If the product that you're distributing is that good then you should be first partaker of health and wellness exemplified and manifested in your life.

As a man many times we refuse to go and get a checkup to see what is going on in our bodies so we continue on as though everything is fine. I personally know an individual that has not had a check-up in over 30 years. Likewise at one time I was stubborn and allowed my pride to get in the way and hadn't had a check-up in about 10 years or more. I say especially to the men, men go get you a check-up to find out what's going on in your body. You may think you are healthy and may even feel healthy but until you know what's going on in your body you're playing Russian roulette with your health. Sickness and diseases doesn't just instantly appear in your body something has been lingering for a while and it finally manifested for you to see.

This could have been prevented or at the least controlled before it turned into something catastrophic or stage 4 cancers. Your blood work will tell the truth of what's really going on in your body. Don't wait until it's too late and you need a miracle or a miracle cure to reverse your health.

I give God the glory for the many checkups I've had in the last 2 years and the amazing and glaring reports I've received from the doctors about my health. I remember one checkup I got along with extensive blood work done and had to go back in a couple of weeks to get the results and two doctors said to me *"Mr. Jones you are in great physical health, your health is so good, out of all my clients I've seen today you are the best. I wish all my clients were in good health like you. Mr. Jones we're trying to find something wrong with you lol, what do you do?"* My response was Praise the Lord, I take Moringa have you ever heard of it? His response was no I haven't but bring me some information on it.

Moringa Over Medicine

Also, another time I went to get a checkup and had blood work done and went back 2 weeks later for my results the doctor told me, *"Mr. Jones you're as healthy as a horse. You're my inspiration for today. Your results look wonderful keep up the great work."* I give God the glory for keeping me in great health and also for his creation Moringa Oleifera that I take on a daily basis. I use to suffer with high cholesterol and low energy but both of those are things of the past. I give God glory that I am probably in as close to perfect health as is humanly possible and I don't even get what many call the common cold nor do I contract the flu during flu season. Moringa Oleifera helps to keep my immune system strong, fight off free radicals and supplies my body with all the essential nutrients needed in this one amazing product. We are first partakers of this product and it has done amazing things in our health and we know that it will likewise bring assistance to you to help to create a new you today the Moringa way.

"There is no money in treating healthy people from a physician standpoint."

1

Sickness In America

"America is sicker than ever because she has blindly turned her will over to medicine without reasoning if medicine is the best option."

When we behold the statistics of sickness and disease in America it baffles the imagination. Here we are in the richest nation in the world and yet one of the sickest nation in the world. People are on more medication now than they have ever been and the sad reality is that individuals are not on just one or two medications but in some case these individuals are taking 5, 10 and 15 different medications at once.

The sad reality is that when one individual may go to see another Doctor about their condition their new physician ask them in unbelief *"why are you taking ALL this medication?"* It seems as if Doctors don't care anymore or

Moringa Over Medicine

they're just prescribing whatever they think will alleviate the cause without any real diagnosis.

Sickness in America is real and it's getting worse because now medication has become a new cash register for money hungry Physicians. It has been noted that *"Americans Spent a Record Amount on Medicine in 2015. In 2015, the U.S. spent **$325 billion** on prescription drug expenditure in the United States according to the Statistics Portal Statistics and Studies from more than 22,500 Sources."* And this is steady increasing because new drugs are coming out yearly with more and more side effects that's causing adverse reaction with these experimental drugs. It has been estimated that by 2021 spending will be between $400-$600 billion according to a report released by Quintiles IMS.

Sickness in America in on an increase because individuals are believing more in the words of their physicians than ever before without taking the initiative to get a second or even a third opinion before

Moringa Over Medicine

they accept that medication. Americans an people all over it's time to also take personal responsibility for your health because nobody cares about you like you.

Sickness in America is on the rise because as you look at your television you are now seeing one commercial after another that is pushing its medication about what's best for your sickness and disease. You're been influenced to ask your doctor about the latest medicine that you just saw on television that's designed to help your illness.

Sickness in America is on the rise because we have become a society of pharmaceutical drug users that have accepted the propaganda that the medical field knows what's best for you. We have succumbed to the status quo and have simply given in that our physician knows better than we do so we must blindly accept everything they say.

Sickness in America is on the rise because we no longer believe in natural herbs and the benefits that can be derived from their consumption instead of

Moringa Over Medicine

immediately turning to medicine. With such a mindset we will continue to hooray medicine and boo natural remedies simply because we don't understand how they can be beneficial to us. **It's time to make a change.**

Sickness in America will continue to rise if we don't educate ourselves on alternatives and at least take a look and listen to see if we may be missing out indeed on what just might be helpful. The word of God tells us that *"With all thy getting get understanding." Proverbs 4:7b* In other words it's telling us that in life we need to make sure that we get clarity, insight and use some common sense. Doctors don't have all the answers just like no one else does; Doctors die from sickness and disease just like everyone else. If they had all the answers then they would surely keep themselves alive at all cost but sadly this is not true.

Sickness in America will continue to rise because pharmaceutical drugs will continue to be a staple in American assistance. Even the word of God tells us

Moringa Over Medicine

that in the last days drugs will increase according to Revelations 9:21 it states *"Neither repented they of their murders, nor of their sorceries."* The word sorceries in Greek is pronounced pharmakeia and means the use or administering of drugs. The word pharmaceutical comes from this word. Also in Revelations 18:23 it states *"for by thy sorceries (pharmakeia or pharmaceutical) were all nations deceived."* So we see that in the last day's pharmaceutical drugs will play a great part in keeping the nations so drugged up that they will be easily deceived.

- *Americans today need medication to go to sleep at night.*
- *Medication to wake up in the morning.*
- *Medication to take them through the day.*
- *Medication to relax them.*
- *Medication to get them going again.*
- *Medication, medication, and more medication.*

Sickness in American will continue to

Moringa Over Medicine

increase because Americans are just afraid to be without their medication and their hope and faith is more in their medication than even in their God. I've seen cases where individuals could not get their medication but they have seen drastic change for the better in their health while taking Moringa but that still was not convincing enough to continue. At the earliest convenience they immediately got back on medication even though a natural supplement was working just wonderfully. They were afraid and they believe their doctors even over their improved health.

Sickness in America will continue to increase unless we find an alternative that will help to decline what Americans are now experiencing.

- In America we're seeing more people get the flu than ever before.
- In American we're seeing more and more cancer cases than ever before.
- In America we're seeing diabetes cases on the rise.

Moringa Over Medicine

- In America we're seeing more people dealing with hypertension.
- In America we're seeing a rise in Arthritis pains, gout, rheumatism, etc.
- In America we're seeing digestive problems on the rise.
- In America we're seeing obesity and overweight on the rise.
- In America we're seeing more women dealing with menopause.
- In America we're seeing many individuals dealing with chronic fatigue syndrome.
- In America we see people that can't sleep at night because of insomnia.
- In America kids are dealing with attention deficit disorders.
- In America people are dealing with eczema and psoriasis.
- In America people are dealing with depression, stress, anxiety and just overall worrying about life issues.
- In America men are dealing with erectile dysfunction.

Moringa Over Medicine

- In America men are dealing with prostate cancer.
- In America people are using pharmaceutical drugs more and more.

When you hear all these statistic and all the things Americans are dealing with and how sickness in America is affecting our society it's sickening of itself. Our Doctors, the FDA, Medicine, the Pharmaceutical Industry, etc.... are failing us miserably. Sickness in America is on the rise, don't let anyone fool you and it's not getting better but worse.

- What are we to do?
- What is the answer?
- Can we continue to just hope that things will get better?
- Or is it time to seek alternatives?

We believe there are other alternatives to help get rid of Sickness in America.

"Some people are taking 5, 10, 15 different medicines and are still sick with no cure in sight.

2
The Truth About Medicine

"The truth about medicine is that the majority of the time your medication will not cure you but only maintain your condition."

I know an individual that has been on blood pressure medicine for over 20 years with no hope in sight of ever getting off them. Medicine will not cure you but at the most it will only maintain your illness but the long term side effects are toxic at best. *In the 16th century, Paracelsus declared that the only difference between a medicine and a poison was in the dose. All medicines were toxic. It was cure or kill.* Even though much has been discovered since the 16th century there still isn't a medicine today that does not carry various side effects. And the side effect can even include DEATH.

The truth about Medicine is that medicine does help on the surface but the qualifying long term side effects are toxic. A sad reality is that sometimes the effects

Moringa Over Medicine

of the medicine taken can be worse than the disease itself. Let's take another look at the medicine or drugs Vioxx that was introduced to the market in May 1999 and approved by the FDA and available for prescription in the United States. This medicine was one of the worse ever seen that was catastrophic in terms of side effects and deaths. It has been noted that this medicine caused a 140,000 heart attacks. That's enough right there to bring someone to imprisonment for negligence in the lives of humans. This is almost unbelievable that it had to get to this high a number before it was taken off the market. But it doesn't stop there on top of 140,000 heart attacks it resulted in about 60,000 deaths because of this one medicine.

- *I did not say 6 deaths, even that would have been to many.*
- *I did not say 60 deaths, no it doesn't stop there.*
- *I did not say 600 deaths, this would have been tragic.*

Moringa Over Medicine

- *I did not say 6000 deaths, this along would have been catastrophic.*
- *I said 60,000 deaths that came as a result of 1 medicine, 1 pharmaceutical drug that cause havoc on the lives of 60,000 families.*

The truth about medicine is that medicine is here to stay; it's not going anywhere because it's too big of a business and it has created too many lifestyles and incomes. Honey, medicine is here to stay and it will continue to cause havoc in the lives of untold millions.

The truth about medicine is that it's a short term solution to a long term problem. It's not going to make the problem better because it's not going to cure anyone and if it does the cases are few and in between, it simply mask the real problem that needs to be dealt with.

The truth about medicine is that they do come with major health risk and many side effects. And the sad reality is that when new prescriptions are used

Moringa Over Medicine

they have a 1 in 5 chance of causing serious side effects for the user.

The truth about medicine is that as long as there are humans to prescribe it to there will be humans ready to use it for one ailment or another. Sickness and diseases are rampant and the majority of society is suffering from one thing or another. It's sad but very rare to find an individual today that's truly healthy and that doesn't take any kind of medication.

The truth about medicine is that the list of sickness and diseases we're dealing with today range from:

- **High Blood Pressure**
- **Diabetes**
- **High Cholesterol**
- **Arthritis** *(in many forms)*
- **Dementia**
- **Fatigue**
- **Cardiovascular Disease**

Moringa Over Medicine

- Depression
- Headaches
- Fibromyalgia
- Hypothyroidism
- Obesity or Weight Gain
- Cancer
- Kidney Disease
- Liver Disease
- Asthma
- Constipation
- COPD
- Erectile Dysfunction
- Epilepsy
- Ulcerative Colitis
- Hormonal Imbalance
- Hepatitis C
- Sinusitis
- Bronchitis

- **Autism**
- **Lupus**
- **Emphysema**
- **Cerebral Palsy**
- **Blood Disorders**
- **Flu**
- **Stroke**
- **Malaria**
- **Hepatitis B**
- **Tuberculosis**
- **ADHD**
- **Chronic Fatigue Syndrome**
- **Heart Disease**
- **Autoimmune Disease**
- **Psoriasis or Eczema**
- **Or Hundreds of Other Diseases...**

Because we're dealing with so many various diseases the medical industry are

Moringa Over Medicine

constantly coming up with various medicines to combat these diseases. But they haven't come up with one medicine that doesn't bring along with it a list of adverse side effects.

I've said before that medicine does have its place in such situations as when an individual has been in a car accident and need medicine for immediate medical attention to save one's life, or for a life threating situation. I believe that God put medicine here for such cases as these and also because it's the only solution that many will look to for health and wellness.

The truth about medicine is that instead of individuals getting better people are still:

- **Obese and overweight.**
- **Dealing with Hypertension.**
- **Dealing with Diabetes.**
- **Dealing with Alzheimer and Dementia.**
- **Dealing with Lupus.**
- **Dealing with Arthritis.**

Moringa Over Medicine

- **Dealing with Heart Disease.**
- **Dealing with Chronic Fatigue Syndrome.**
- **Dealing with Autoimmune Disease.**
- **Dealing with Cancer.**
- **Dealing with 100's of other diseases.**

The professionals and pharmaceutical companies can say all they like that medicine is helping individuals and things are getting better. Well here are facts:

- *In 2010 Americans spent $253.1 Billion dollars on prescription drugs.*
- *In 2011 Americans spent $258.8 Billion dollars on prescription drugs.*
- *In 2012 Americans spent $259.2 Billion dollars on prescription drugs.*
- *In 2013 Americans spent $265.2 Billion dollars on prescription drugs.*
- *In 2014 Americans spent $298 Billion dollars on prescription drugs.*

Moringa Over Medicine

- *In 2015 Americans spent $324.5 Billion dollars on prescription drugs.*
- *In 2016 Americans spent $328.6 Billion dollars on prescription drugs.*
- *In 2017 Americans spent $338.1 Billion dollars on prescription drugs.*
- *In 2018 Americans spent $360.2 Billion dollars so far on prescription drugs.*
- *Information is derived from "The Statistic Portal"*

Pharmaceutical medicine is one of the most profitable businesses there is and these companies will never run out of customers. As long as sickness and disease is around billions and billions of dollars will be made by these companies. Vioxx paid out 5 billion dollars to plaintiffs and around 2 billion dollars in legal fees but they still walked away with about 4 billion dollars after killing around 60,000 people.

The truth about medicine is they're not really looking for a cure just new medicines to maintain your disease. If

Moringa Over Medicine

they cure you then there will be no further need for developing new drugs. No they don't want a medicine to cure you but one that will drag you along until some other disease develops in your body and you need another medicine to sustain you for a little longer.

The truth about medicine is that medicine is simply a bandage on a big wound that will never heal up but will simply cover it up.

- How can you take medicine for hypertension (high blood pressure) for 20 + years and your blood pressure never stabilizes?
- How can you take medicine for diabetes for 20 + years and your body still does not produce enough insulin?
- How can you take medicine for high cholesterol for 20 + years and still have fatty deposits in your blood vessels still causing high cholesterol?

Moringa Over Medicine

- How can you take medicine for arthritis for years and still have inflammation ravaging your body with no signs of curing you?
- How can you take medicine for dementia that the medical industry says can neither slow it down nor cure it but only ease some of the symptoms? Medicine that gives no future hope for the users?
- And time would fail me to tell about medicine for depression, headaches, cardiovascular diseases, chronic fatigue syndrome, fibromyalgia, hypothyroidism, obesity, kidney disease, liver disease, asthma, copd, erectile dysfunction, epilepsy, ulcerative colitis, hepatitis c, sinusitis, and hundreds of other diseases that never see a cure and give no real future hope for the users?

The future hope for medicine for the human body is bleak, spending will increase and more deaths will occur!

Moringa Over Medicine

"Moringa Oleifera is a miracle plant that has so many benefits that it's almost unbelievable that one plant can do so much."

3
The Truth About Moringa Oleifera

"And God said, Behold, I have given you every herb bearing seed, which is upon the face of all the earth, and every tree, in the which is the fruit of a tree yielding seed; to you it shall be for meat."

There is a plant or tree called the Moringa Oleifera and it's the greatest plant on the planet. You may ask what makes this plant so great. Well, when God created the Moringa Oleifera tree he placed within that tree all the nutrients that our body need in a single plant. There is no other plant on the planet that can be given that right but Moringa Oleifera. It's amazing the nutrients that it contains, Moringa has:

- **3 times the Potassium in bananas.**
- **7 times the Vitamin-C as in oranges.**
- **25 times the Iron in spinach.**

Moringa Over Medicine

- 4 times the Calcium in milk.
- 4 times the Vitamin A in Carrots.
- 46 + Antioxidants
- 36 Anti-Inflammatory Compounds
- 90 + Nutrients.
- 18 + Amino Acids
- 8 Essential Amino Acids — the one your body cannot survive without but cannot manufacture on its own.
- 20 times more Vitamin E than Tofu.
- 2 times more Protein than Eggs.
- 10 times more Vitamin E than Nuts.
- **Moringa contains Omega-3, 6, & 9.**
- **Vitamins:** A, B1, B2, B3, B5, B6, B7, B8, B9 B12, C, D, E, K, Choline, Flavonoids.
- **Minerals:** Calcium, Magnesium,

Moringa Over Medicine

Phosphorus, Potassium, Sodium, Sulfur, Cobalt, Copper, Aluminum, Arsenic, Barium, Beryllium, Boron, Bromine, Carbon, Iodine, Iron, Manganese, Selenium, Zinc, Cerium, Cesium, Chromium, Dysprosium, Erbium, Europium, Gadolinium, Gallium, Germanium, Gold, Hafnium, Holmium, Hydrogen, Lanthanum, Lithium, Lutetium, Molybdenum, Neodymium, Nickel, Niobium, Nitrogen, Oxygen, Praseodymium, Rhenium, Rubidium, Samarium, Scandium, Silica, Silver, Strontium, Tantalum, Terbium, Thulium, Tin, Titanium, Vanadium, Ytterbium, Yttrium, Zirconium

- **All 8 Essential Amino Acids:** Isoleucine, Leucine, Lysine, Methionine, Phenylalanine, Threonine, Tryptophan, Valine.

- **10 Additional Amino Acids:** Alanine, Arganine, Aspartic Acid, Cystine, Glutamine, Glycine, Histidine, Proline, Serine, Tyrosine.

Moringa Over Medicine

Other Beneficial Nutrients: Chlorophyll, Carotenoids, Cytokinins, Plant Sterols, Polyphenols, and more. **All in 1 plant.**

There is no other plant on the planet that can give your body these **nutrients in 1 single plant.** Many times we experience various sickness and diseases because we are deficient in vitamins and minerals. When you're lacking essential nutrients then your body begins to work against you instead of with you.

Moringa is the most powerful superfood ever discovered by mankind. For thousands of years it has been a remedy for mankind as far back as the Ayurvedic medicine one of the world's oldest medical methods that originated in India over 3,000 years ago and still practiced today. Our objective in bringing to the forefront Moringa in our Western society is to inform individuals of the benefits that are derived from the consumption of

Moringa Over Medicine

this amazing plant. It is a plant that supplies our bodies with all the essential nutrients for a healthy body. This eliminates the widespread cost of having to purchase various supplements to provide your body with the necessary nutrients for wholeness and wellness. One can spend a small fortune trying to purchase various vitamin supplements to make up the whole of what's needed for a daily supplement. However, with Moringa you have it all in 1 plant.

We encourage individuals to take Moringa for 2 reasons:

1. *Prevention of sickness and disease.*
2. *Restoration of your body to meet your health and wellness needs.*

These are the main reasons why one would add Moringa Oleifera to their daily dietary supplement. We will delve into these two reasons and how God's Superfood can aid, help, and assist mankind in keeping his temple (body) in tip top shape or restoring it to a healthy state. There is no reason why you have to live a life of sickness and disease when God's has already supplied mankind with the remedy for good health. Mankind just has to be obedient to learn and apply what God says about Moringa and how he designed this plant to help our bodies rid itself of toxic things that can hurt us. As well as how Moringa can supply our bodies with the essential nutrients to maintain good health and help reverse bad health.

PREVENTION OF SICKNESS AND DISEASE

Seeing a sick body restored back to health is a wonderful thing. However, what's better than restoration is a body that remains healthy consistently. No one wants to encounter sickness even if good health or healing is right around the corner. The best method is **PREVENTION** at all cost. One of the great things we've found about Moringa is that it has within it what it takes to get and maintain a **HEALTHY BODY**. Moringa is the greatest weapon against prevention of sickness and disease. Having Moringa in your system is like always having a doctor on hand because once it gets in your system it works around the clock 24/7 and 365 days a year.

With all the nutrients in Moringa it has been discovered that this amazing plant has the highest protein ratio of any plant analyzed so far. With such inherited protein it's an absolute that your body will not only survive but thrive as every cell in your body is impacted with the highest protein available today in plant form. Because our bodies use protein to repair and build tissue Moringa is an important building block of our body functions. With such an infusion of essential proteins your body will take care of itself as Moringa both prevent the occurrence of disease as well as slow down the rate or frequency of disease.

Moringa is a product when used on a consistent basis has the power to intervene and deter any evidence of disease or sickness. It has the ability to eliminate problems at the source, thereby preventing the occurrence of an issue. Moringa's aim is to empower your body to be able to sustain itself and thereby reduce the risk of developing diseases.

A healthy body honors and glorifies God; a sick body deprives you of use and dishonors God. The scripture says, *"What? know ye not that your body is the temple of the Holy Ghost which is in you, which ye have of God, and ye are not your own? For ye are bought with a price: therefore glorify God in your body, and in your spirit, which are God's"* 1 Corinthians 6:19-20

The key to a healthy life is **PREVENTION** not **RESTORATION.**

The act of restoration only comes because you have failed in prevention. The one way to prevent diseases is by maintaining good health and keeping a proper assessment of what is going on in your body. **Moringa Oleifera does this for you.**

RESTORATION OF THE BODY TO HEALTH AND WELLNESS

In our society we have millions of individuals that are suffering with various diseases and sickness. From high blood pressure, diabetes, cardiovascular disease, obesity, fatigue, etc.... and it's taking its toll on our society. Individuals that are dealing with these diseases have one thing in mind and that is either healing for their body or restoring their body back to health.

Restoration is needed when you have failed at prevention and now you need to get your body back to health. Well, Moringa Oleifera is also an excellent restorer to health by resupplying your

Moringa Over Medicine

body with the essential nutrients that it has been deprived of and thereby sickness has taken the advantage of your deprivation. There is no need to give up all hope and throw in the towel; Moringa is here to rescue you as God's Superfood.

Moringa Oleifera can aid and assist you to return your body to a normal or healthy condition as God designed it to do. Moringa gets to the source of the problem and helps your body to heal itself as the missing nutrients helps your body to fight off toxins that make it sick while at the same time strengthening your body functions by giving it new life as you absorb the miracle working power of Moringa.

There are several ways Moringa does this to help restore health and wellness to your body.

1. *It detoxifies your body.*
2. *It removes the parasites out of your body.*

Moringa Over Medicine

3. *It builds up your immune system.*
4. *It fights off free radicals with its rich amount of antioxidants.*
5. *It reduces inflammation in the body.*
6. *It protects the cardiovascular system.*
7. *It helps to support the brain health.*
8. *It helps to protect the liver.*
9. *It helps to protect the kidneys.*
10. *Moringa contains antimicrobial and antibacterial properties.*
11. *Moringa helps to reduce stress.*
12. *It helps to support a healthy digestive system.*
13. *It helps to maintain strong and healthy bones.*
14. *Moringa helps to balance your hormones.*
15. *Moringa protects and nourishes the skin.*

16. *Moringa contains 90+ nutrients to meet your physical needs.*

17. *Moringa contains 36 anti-inflammatory compounds.*

18. *Moringa contains 46 antioxidants.*

19. *Moringa contains 8 essential amino acids which your body needs but cannot produce.*

20. *Moringa contains phytonutrients like zeatin, quercetin, beta-sistosterol, caffeeoylquinic acid and kaempferol.*

21. *Moringa boosts energy level naturally.*

Moringa is known by over 100 names in various parts of the world and is now becoming very popular in the United States. In 2008, the National Institute of Health called Moringa Oleifera the **"plant of the year."** Also, according to the ORAC, Moringa scored 157,000, topping all the other antioxidants superfoods on the market today. Including such superfoods as Acai berries, Green tea, Blueberries, Dark Chocolate, Ginger, Kale, Matcha, Spirulina, Turmeric, Garlic, Goji berries, Pomegranates, Red Wine, Etc.

There's no better or more qualified plant today for Prevention or Restoring your health back to normal. Prevention is the key and Restoration is both a process and a journey and Moringa Oleifera is God's Superfood that will bring life back into your body.

The sickness and diseases that you're experiencing are a result of **"A Deficiency of Vitamins and Minerals."** When your body does not have the nutrients that it needs then it cannot function as it should. Your body becomes deficient in vitamins and minerals when it doesn't obtain or absorb the amount of vitamins and minerals it requires. Your body must have different amount of each vitamin and mineral in order to stay healthy and when the required amount is

Moringa Over Medicine

not there then you've become deficient in those vitamins and minerals.

In this chapter we will give you a list of diseases and the deficiency of vitamins and minerals that contribute to these diseases:

ASTHMA: A person that has asthma is deficient in such nutrients as: **Vitamin D, Vitamin E, Vitamin C, Polyunsaturated fatty acids (Omega 3 & 6), Selenium, Zinc, Magnesium, Manganese, Flavonoids, Vitamin B12, Folate, Vitamin B6,** just to name a few. But if you will notice from the list of nutrients contained in Moringa Oleifera it has all these nutrients in this 1 plant.

ERECTILE DYSFUNCTION: A person that is experiencing erectile dysfunction is deficient in such nutrients as: **Vitamin D, Manganese, Magnesium, Vitamin B3, Folate, Vitamin B12, Amino Acids, Zinc,** just to name a few. But if you will notice from the list of nutrients contained in

Moringa Over Medicine

Moringa Oleifera it has all these nutrients in this 1 plant.

KIDNEY DISEASE: A person that's experiencing kidney disease is deficient in such nutrients as: **Vitamin B Complex, Iron, Vitamin D, Vitamin C, and Calcium,** just to name a few. But if you will notice from the list of nutrients contained in Moringa Oleifera it has all these nutrients in this 1 plant.

LIVER DISEASE: A person that's experiencing liver disease is deficient in such nutrients as: **Antioxidants, Zinc, Selenium, Beta-carotene, Vitamin D, Vitamin A, and Magnesium,** just to name a few. But if you will notice from the list of nutrients contained in Moringa Oleifera it has all these nutrients in this 1 plant.

EPILEPSY: A person that's experiencing epilepsy is deficient in such nutrients as: **Vitamin B6, Calcium, Carnitine, Vitamin D, Vitamin E, Folate, Magnesium, Selenium, Vitamin B1,**

Moringa Over Medicine

Vitamin B12, Sodium, just to name a few. But if you will notice from the list of nutrients contained in Moringa Oleifera it has all these nutrients in this 1 plant

ULCERATIVE COLITIS: A person that's experiencing ulcerative colitis is deficient in such nutrients as: **Vitamin B12, Iron, Vitamin D, Vitamin K, Folate, Selenium, Zinc, Vitamin B6 and Vitamin B1,** just to name a few. But if you will notice from the list of nutrients contained in Moringa Oleifera it has all these nutrients in this 1 plant.

GOUT: A person that's experiencing gout is deficient in such nutrients as: **Calcium, Vitamin D, Potassium, and Magnesium,** just to name a few. But if you will notice from the list of nutrients contained in Moringa Oleifera it has all these nutrients in this 1 plant.

HORMONAL IMBALANCE: A person that is experiencing hormonal imbalance is deficient in such nutrients as: **Vitamin C, Vitamin E, Calcium, Magnesium,**

Moringa Over Medicine

Vitamin B Complex, just to name a few. But if you will notice from the list of nutrients contained in Moringa Oleifera it has all these nutrients in this 1 plant.

STROKE: A person that is experiencing a STROKE is deficient in such nutrients as: **Iron, Vitamin B12, Fiber, Vitamin D, Vitamin C, Folate and Antioxidants,** just to name a few. . But if you will notice from the list of nutrients contained in Moringa Oleifera it has all these nutrients in this 1 plant.

ANEMIA: A person that is experiencing anemia is deficient in such nutrients as: **Iron, Vitamin B12, Folate, and Vitamin C,** just to name a few. But if you will notice from the list of nutrients contained in Moringa Oleifera it has all these nutrients in this 1 plant.

CONSTIPATION: A person that is experiencing constipation is deficient in such nutrients as: **Vitamin B12, Vitamin B1, Folate, Vitamin B5, Vitamin C, Potassium, Magnesium and Fiber,** just to name a few. But if you will notice from the list of nutrients contained in Moringa Oleifera it has all these nutrients in this 1 plant.

SARCOIDOSIS: A person that is experiencing sarcoidosis is deficient in such nutrients as: **Vitamin A, Vitamin C, Vitamin E, Vitamin B-Complex, Magnesium, Calcium, Zinc, Selenium and Omega-3 Fatty Acids,**

HIGH BLOOD PRESSURE: Take for example a person that has high blood pressure they're deficient in such nutrients as: **Potassium, Magnesium, Omega 3 fats, Calcium and Coenzyme Q10 that acts as an antioxidant in our cells,** just to name a few. But if you will notice from the list of nutrients contained in Moringa Oleifera it has all these nutrients in this 1 plant.

ARTHRITIS: A person that has arthritis is deficient in such nutrients as: **Vitamin D, Folate, Calcium, and Omega 3 fatty Acids,** just to name a few. Also, if you will notice that Moringa Oleifera has all these essential nutrients in this one plant.

DIABETES: A person that has diabetes is deficient in such nutrients as: **Vitamin B12, Vitamin D, Vitamin E, Magnesium, Zinc, Vitamin B6, Folate, Vitamin C and Antioxidants,** just to name a few. However, if you will notice from the list of nutrients in Moringa Oleifera all these are contained in this 1 plant.

HIGH CHOLESTEROL: A person that has high cholesterol is most of the time deficient in such nutrients as: **Vitamin B12, Iron, Biotin, Inositol, Chromium, Copper, Manganese, Potassium, Vanadium, and Zinc,** just to name a few. However, if you will notice from the list of nutrients in Moringa Oleifera all these are contained in this 1 plant.

DEMENTIA: A person that is dealing with Dementia is deficient in such nutrients as: **Vitamin B1, Vitamin E, Phosphatidylserine (PS) (is a phospholipid-a fat containing phosphorus), Vitamin B12, Folate, Zinc,**

just to name a few. But if you will notice from the list of nutrients in Moringa Oleifera all these are contained in this 1 plant.

FATIGUE (Tiredness or lack of Energy): A person that is experiencing fatigue or lack of energy is deficient in a variety of nutrients such as: **Vitamin B12, Folate, Vitamin D, Iron, Magnesium, and Potassium,** just to name a few. But if you will notice from the list of nutrients in Moringa Oleifera all these are contained in this 1 plant.

CARDIOVASCULAR DISEASE: A person that's experiencing cardiovascular disease is deficient in such nutrients as: **Vitamin D, Coenzyme Q10, Iron, Vitamin B1(Thiamine), Amino Acids, Folate, Flavonoids, Vanadium, Vitamin E,** just to name a few. But if you will notice from the list of nutrients in Moringa Oleifera all these are contained in this 1 plant.

DEPRESSION: A person that's dealing

with experiencing depression is deficient in such nutrients as: **Omega-3 Fatty Acids, Vitamin D, Magnesium, Vitamin B Complex, Folate, Amino Acids, Iron, Zinc, Iodine, Selenium,** just to name a few. But if you will notice from the list of nutrients in Moringa Oleifera all these are contained in this 1 plant.

HEADACHES: A person that's experiencing various kinds of headaches from migraine to regular headaches are deficient in such nutrients as: **Vitamin D, Riboflavin, Coenzyme Q10, Folate, Vitamin B Complex, Vitamin E, Magnesium, Iron,** just to name a few. But if you will notice from the list of nutrients in Moringa Oleifera all these are contained in this 1 plant.

FIBROMYALGIA: A person that's experiencing fibromyalgia is deficient in such nutrients as: **Vitamin D, Magnesium, Iron, Amino Acids, Vitamin B12, and Calcium,** just to name a few. But if you will notice from the list of nutrients in Moringa Oleifera all these are contained in this 1 plant.

HYPOTHYROIDISM: A person that's experiencing hypothyroidism is deficient in such nutrients as: **Iodine, Vitamin B Complex, Selenium, Zinc, Vitamin D, Tyrosine, Vitamin A, Iron,** just to name a few. But if you will notice from the list of nutrients in Moringa Oleifera all these are contained in this 1 plant.

WEIGHT LOSS: When dealing with obesity or overweight you need to make sure that you're getting the essential nutrients for your physical body. Weight loss is more than just losing weight; you want to make sure that you're healthy while losing that weight. Research has proven that individuals that obtain the lowest amount of nutrients are gaining the most weight. Most individuals are deficient in such nutrients as: **Iron, Vitamin D, Vitamin B Complex, Magnesium, Vitamin A, Iodine, Vitamin C, Calcium,** just to name a few. But if you will notice from the list of nutrients in

Moringa Over Medicine

Moringa Oleifera all these are contained in this 1 plant.

LUPUS: A person dealing with lupus is deficient in such nutrients as: **Vitamin D, Vitamin E, Zinc, Vitamin A, Vitamin B Complex, Vitamin C, Magnesium, Iron, Omega 3 fatty acids, Antioxidants, Calcium,** just to name a few. But if you will notice from the list of nutrients in Moringa Oleifera all these are contained in this 1 plant.

CANCER: A person dealing with cancer has a broader spectrum of things going on but making sure that your body has the essential nutrients can play a great part in recovery. Some research has also revealed that certain forms of cancer are more widespread among some regions where there is great nutrient deficiency. Some of the nutrients you will need to include in your daily diet are: **Vitamin D, Vitamin K, Iodine, Magnesium, Selenium, Vitamin B Complex, Vitamin C, Iron, Folate, Vitamin A, Coenzyme Q10,** just to name a few. But if you will

Moringa Over Medicine

notice from the list of nutrients in Moringa Oleifera all these are contained in this 1 plant.

While your body is supplied with all the nutrients to combat these diseases you're also taking in an awesome supply of such things as:

- **46 + Antioxidants**
- **36 Anti-Inflammatories**
- **Moringa contains Omega 3, 6, & 9.**
- **18 + Amino Acids**
- **8 Essential Amino Acids — the one your body cannot survive without but cannot manufacture on its own.**
- **Moringa contains Silymarin an Antioxidant that's great for liver problems.**
- **Moringa contains ZEATIN, which regulates cell division and growth, plus it has ant-aging properties that delay cell aging. The ZEATIN**

in Moringa has several thousand times more in it than any other plant on the planet.

Moringa is the most powerful superfood that God has ever allowed man to discover to date. It is one product that contains no fillers, additives, preservatives, etc.... Therefore, when you have Moringa you have one natural supplement that covers many things your body requires and needs instead of buying several supplements that can be very expensive. There is no other plant on the planet that carries a more compacted profile of nutrients in one product.

Even if you're eating a properly balanced meal your meal is still deficient in vitamins and minerals because our soils today are depleted by the rigorous growth methods that cause our food to lack the essential nutrients needed for our bodies. Yet, Moringa is the only plant that can provide your body with all the nutrients that's needed on a daily basis. Moringa Oleifera is often called "The

Moringa Over Medicine

Miracle Tree" because of the enormous health benefits that one derives from using it. This plant has a long history of success according to India's age old tradition known as Ayurveda who for centuries used Moringa Oleifera as a healing plant.

Our Moringa sold and distributed at "Eden Wellness Moringa" is superior quality, superior grade, organically grown, 100% pure, non-polluted, high potent, USDA Organic, caffeine free, non-gmo, gluten free, all natural, chemical free & pesticide free. We have the finest leaves, seeds, etc. harvested in the right stage.

So there you have the truth about Moringa Oleifera and why it's called the greatest plant on the planet because no other plant can give your body what it needs in 1 plant. **Knowledge is a powerful thing.**

"And God saw everything that he had made, and, behold, it was very good." Genesis 1:31a

4
Moringa Over Medicine

"If the pharmaceutical industry came up with cures for all the major diseases they would be out of business."

The pharmaceutical industry is not interested in a medicinal cure, because a cure would put them out of business.

The individuals that sell and distribute Moringa Oleifera have one main goal and that is health and wellness for all.

The pharmaceutical industry is all about the money and without medical care most individuals would not be able to afford medicine. And those without medical care are just down right pitiful.

The individuals that sell and distribute Moringa Oleifera sell and distribute Moringa at an affordable price so that the ordinary person can afford it.

Moringa Over Medicine

The pharmaceutical industries are selling and distributing medicines that have numerous side effects and some of those side effects include death.

The Moringa Oliefera industry sells and distributes moringa a product that has no side effects and no deaths recorded.

Medicine is a man-made product created in a lab, designed by man, formulated by man with all the side effects of man's manipulation.

The Moringa Oleifera plant is a tree created by the Creator and given for the aid, assistance and help of man. *"He causeth the grass to grow for the cattle, and herb for the service (the aid, assistance, and help) of man: that he may bring forth food out of the earth." Psalms 104:14*

Medicine from a prescribed perspective is defined as a pharmaceutical **drug** that legally requires

Moringa Over Medicine

a medical prescription to be dispensed.

Moringa Oleifera is **a plant** that is called the drumstick tree that has been used for thousands of years for its medicinal properties and health benefits.

Medicine is a **drug** which is defined as a chemical that is given to people in order to treat or prevent an illness.

Moringa is a **food** and a **vegetable** that's rich in nutrients. It's a food just like kale, spinach, collard greens, etc…

Medicine is **chemical based** and created in a lab. A chemical is defined as a compound or substance that has been purified or prepared, especially artificially.

Moringa Oleifera is a plant **free of chemicals** and that is comprised of 90+ Nutrients, 46 + Antioxidants, 36 Anti-Inflammatory Compounds, 18 + Amino Acids and 8 Essential Amino Acids — the

Moringa Over Medicine

ones your body cannot survive without but cannot manufacture on its own.

Medicine is FDA approved as a drug that can treat, cure or prevent a disease, even though we rarely if ever see diseases cured.

Moringa Oleifera is a plant that has to be stated in accordance with the FDA as *"These statements have not been evaluated by the Food & Drug Administration. This product is not intended to treat, diagnose, cure or prevent any disease."*

Medicine can only be prescribed by a FDA approved pharmaceutical company that has been given a patent for that drug.

Moringa Oleifera cannot be patent by any company and does not have to be approved by the FDA.

Medicine causes other sickness and diseases in the body by all the side effects associated with it. While it's supposed to

Moringa Over Medicine

help one thing it's affecting other parts of your body.

Moringa Oleifera is considered a superfood that builds up your immune system and fights off free radicals.

Medicine is toxic and creates toxins in your body. There is such a thing as Drug toxicity and it has been a common and significant health problem for many.

Moringa Oleifera removes toxins from your body and detoxifies your body as well as removes parasites from your body.

Medicine can be poisonous or harmful when taken wrongly and can even cause death in many cases.

Moringa Oleifera is neither poisonous nor harmful even when taken in large doses. At the most it will upset the stomach in large doses.

Moringa Over Medicine

Medicine is a cash cow for pharmaceutical companies and therefore whenever it has finally been taken off the market because of great side effects like heart attacks, deaths, etc... it has already made millions or billions of dollars for the pharmaceutical companies.

Moringa Oleifera is no cash cow for this industry and millions or billions are not made as a result. Because the individuals that sells it are more concern with health and wellness than riches and wealth.

Medicine is promoted through million dollar television ads paid to actors to pose as users of the medicine.

Moringa Oleifera have no million dollar ads and no millions to pay actors to promote or market their products. They prefer to use users of the products first and foremost.

Medicine kills around a 125,000 people

Moringa Over Medicine

each year as a result of the side effects of these medicines.

Moringa Oleifera has no recorded deaths in over 3000 years of use and no side effects.

Medicine is sold more than ever before yet people are sicker than ever before.

Moringa Oleifera is giving people their life back and helping them to live a better quality of life.

Medicines in the form of antibiotics are being prescribed at over a hundred million per year but people are still getting sick.

Moringa Oleifera contains both antimicrobial and antibacterial properties.

Medicine does not contain the natural nutrients that your body needs without the adverse side effects.

Moringa Over Medicine

Moringa Oleifera contains phytonutrients like zeatin, quercetin, beta-sistosterol, caffeeoylquinic acid and kaempferol.

Medicine does not contain the 90 + nutrients that your body needs to meet your physical needs.

Moringa Oleifera contains 90 + nutrients to meet your physical needs.

Medicine in no form reduces inflammation without the possibility of adverse side effects.

Moringa Oleifera reduces the inflammation in the body without side effects.

Some medicines can harm both your liver and kidneys with the adverse side effects associated with these medicines.

Moringa Oleifera protects the liver and kidneys as a result of the minerals that

Moringa Over Medicine

are derived from this plant.

Medicine causes other medical problems to arise in your life. Medicines only suppress the symptoms they do not treat the cause of the problem.

Moringa Oleifera has antibacterial, antifungal, antimicrobial, properties that can help combat infections and get or keep you on the road to health and wellness.

Medicine can cause the body to become imbalance because of the side effects and when the body is imbalance it's more susceptible and open to other diseases.

Moringa Oleifera keeps the body balance because the body now has the essential nutrients needed to protect it and now your body works with you instead of against you.

Medicines can weaken your immune

system or defense system and a weaken systems invites physical troubles.

Moringa Oleifera strengthens your immune system or defense system and a strong immune system means a strong physical body.

Medicine makes your body more acidic because of the toxins and therefore your body is more susceptible to sickness and diseases.

Moringa Oleifera makes your body more alkaline and when your body is more alkaline then you're on the path to health and wellness.

It's time for each individual to take personal responsibility for their own health. It's not God's responsibility, your doctors, your friends, your leaders, etc… It's YOURS! It's time to learn what you need to know and apply what you've learned to have Health Over Sickness.

"Moringa Oleifera is God's Superfood, it's more than just a vitamin or mineral supplement, and it's a way of life."

5
God's Spiritual Superfood

"And God said, Behold, I have given you every herb bearing seed, which is upon the face of all the earth, and every tree, in the which is the fruit of a tree yielding seed; to you it shall be for meat."

When the Creator made the heavens and the earth it was his objective that mankind should live off of the herbs of the field. The trees were to be the food that mankind was to eat on a daily basis. All of the food in the Garden of Eden was considered God's Spiritual Superfoods before the fall. Every plant was life, every fruit was full of nutrients and Adam and Eve could live off of the fruit of the trees.

However, when mankind ate of the forbidden fruit then the ground became cursed as it is stated *"And unto Adam he said, Because thou hast hearkened unto the voice of thy wife, and hast eaten of the tree, of which I commanded thee, saying, Thou shalt not eat of it: cursed is the ground for thy sake; in sorrow shalt thou eat of it all the days of thy life. Thorns also and thistles shall it bring forth to thee; and thou shalt eat the herb of the field." Genesis 3:17b*

Now that God's food supply in its entirety for mankind is no longer Spiritual Superfoods now man has to browse to know what's harmful and what's healthy. Now there are plants that can kill and plants that can heal. There are many plants in the earth today that's good for our bodies and these plants can change your health from sickness to wellness from disease to wholeness.

Since the fall of mankind God has used different method and means to get man back to a state of health and wellness. He has informed them about what foods to eat and what foods to abstain from. What foods were clean and which foods were unclean. He has given man a list in His holy word to try and change man's mindset for a better life. He just asks man to obey his list of eating instructions and man would be better off.

Moringa Over Medicine

The list of natural herbs that God has given mankind to aid and assist him to remain in health and wellness is vast. There are many herbs that are now labeled as just Superfoods and they are working wonderfully in helping in the way of prevention or restoration. Some of these Superfoods that we're familiar with today were rated according to their ORAC value. *ORAC stands for Oxygen Radical Absorbance Capacity. It's a lab test that attempts to quantify the "total antioxidant capacity" (TAC) of a food by placing a sample of the food in a test tube, along with certain molecules that generate free radical activity and certain other molecules that are vulnerable to oxidation (Scientific America)* **rating are:**

- Moringa Oleifera – 157,000
- Dried Thyme – 157,380
- Matcha Tea – 134,800
- Cinnamon (Ground) – 131,420
- Turmeric (Ground) – 127,068
- Vanilla Beans – 122,400
- Sage (Ground) – 119,929

Moringa Over Medicine

- Black Tea Powder — 112,800
- Acai (fruit pulp/skin powder) — 102,700
- Dried Parsley — 73,670
- Nutmeg (Ground) — 69,640
- Dried Basil — 61,063
- Cumin Seed — 50,372
- Baking Chocolate — 49,944
- White Pepper — 40,700
- Ginger (Ground) — 39,041
- Goji Berries — 25,300
- Spirulina Powder — 24,000
- Chili Powder — 23,636
- Paprika — 21,932
- Dark Chocolate — 20,816
- Black Raspberries — 19,220
- Pecans — 17,940
- Chokeberry (Raw) — 16,062
- Ginger Root (Raw) — 14,840
- Elderberries (Raw) — 14,697
- Fresh Oregano — 13,970
- Walnuts — 13,541
- Raisins (Golden Seedless) — 10,450
- Artichokes — 9,416
- Kidney Beans — 8,606

Moringa Over Medicine

- Dried Plums — 8,059
- Pomegranate (Raw) — 4,479
- Red Apples — 4,275
- Red Wine — 3,600
- Broccoli Boiled — 2,160
- Avocado (Raw) — 1,922
- Spinach (Raw) — 1,513
- Green Tea — 1,240
- Fresh Kiwi — 862

As you can see in this list Moringa Oleifera tops all the Superfoods and many by a landslide. We've chosen to sell and distribute Moringa Oleifera out of all of God's Superfood because nothing compares with it in nutritional value. This is as close to a perfect food as possible to get. Behold this amazing food.

Information content starting from page (91-114) was contributed by Sandra Toliver. Her body of knowledge about Moringa Oleifera and nutrients are amazing and I'm honored for her contribution in this book.

Moringa Nutritional Benefits-Healthiest Plant on Earth-A Complete Food-All Natural Raw Food

MORINGA'S BENEFITS: are derived from the plant's high concentration of bio-available nutrients. It contains high levels of Vitamin A (beta carotene), Vitamin B1 (Thiamine), Vitamin B2 (Riboflavin), Vitamin B3 (Niacin), Vitamin B6 (Pyridoxine), Vitamin B7 (Biotin), Vitamin B12 (methylcobalamin), Vitamin C (Ascorbic Acid), Vitamin D (Cholecalciferol), Vitamin E (Tocopherol) and Vitamin K.

Vitamin A (beta carotene) is needed by the retina of the eye in the form of a specific metabolite, the light-absorbing molecule retinal. This molecule is absolutely necessary for both scotopic vision and color vision. Vitamin A also functions in a very different role - as an irreversibly oxidized form retinoic acid, which is an important hormone-like growth factor for epithelial and other cells.

Vitamin B1 (thiamine) helps fuel the body by converting blood sugar into energy. It keeps the mucous membranes healthy and is essential for the nervous system and cardiovascular and muscular functions.

Vitamin B2 (riboflavin) is required for a wide variety of cellular processes. Like the other B vitamins, it plays a key role in energy metabolism, and for the metabolism of fats, ketone bodies, carbohydrates, and proteins. It is the central component of the cofactors FAD and FMN, and is therefore required by all "Flavoproteins".

Vitamin B3 (niacin), like all B complex vitamins, is necessary for healthy skin, hair, eyes, and liver. It also helps the nervous system function properly. Niacin helps the body produce sex and stress-related hormones in the adrenal glands and other parts of the body. It is effective in improving circulation and reducing cholesterol levels in the blood.

Vitamin B6 (pyridoxine) is required for the synthesis of the neurotransmitters serotonin and norepinephrine and for myelin formation. Pyridoxine deficiency in adults principally affects the peripheral nerves, skin, mucous membranes, and the blood cell system. In children, the central nervous system (CNS) is also affected. Deficiency can occur in people with uremia, alcoholism, cirrhosis, hyperthyroidism, malabsorption syndromes, congestive heart failure (CHF), and in those taking certain medications.

Vitamin B7 (biotin) has vital metabolic functions. Without biotin as a co-factor, many enzymes do not work properly, and serious complications can occur, including varied diseases of the skin, intestinal tract, and nervous system.

Moringa Over Medicine

Biotin can help address high blood glucose levels in people with type 2 diabetes, and is helpful in maintaining healthy hair and nails, decreasing insulin resistance and improving glucose tolerance, and possibly preventing birth defects. It plays a role in energy metabolism, and has been used to treat alopecia, cancer, Crohn's disease, hair loss, Parkinson's disease, peripheral neuropathy, Rett syndrome, seborrheic dermatitis, and vaginal candidiasis.

Vitamin B12 (Inserted by Dexter L. Jones) (Methyl cobalamin) Methyl cobalamin is the specific form of B12 needed for nervous system health. Vitamin B12 plays an important role in helping the body make red blood cells. Methyl cobalamin is a water-soluble vitamin. The body uses vitamin B12 in energy production and regulation, among other metabolic roles.

Vitamin C (ascorbic acid) is one of the safest and most effective nutrients, experts say. It may not be the cure for the common cold (though it's thought to help prevent more serious complications), but the benefits of vitamin C may include protection against immune system deficiencies, cardiovascular disease, prenatal health problems, eye disease, and wrinkles.

Vitamin D (cholecalciferol) is essential for promoting calcium absorption in the gut and maintaining adequate serum calcium and phosphate concentrations to enable normal mineralization of bone and prevent hypocalcemic tetany. It is also needed for bone growth and bone remodeling by osteoblasts and osteoclasts. Without sufficient vitamin D, bones can become thin, brittle, or misshapen. Vitamin D sufficiency prevents rickets in children and osteomalacia in adults. Together with calcium, vitamin D also helps protect the elderly from osteoporosis. Vitamin D has other roles in human health, including modulation of neuromuscular and immune function and reduction of inflammation.

Vitamin E describes a family of eight antioxidants, four tocopherols and four tocotrienols. alpha-tocopherol (a-tocopherol) is the only form of vitamin E that is actively maintained in the human body and is therefore, the form of vitamin E found in the largest quantities in the blood and tissue. Vitamin E, a fat-soluble vitamin, protects vitamin A and essential fatty acids from oxidation in the body cells and prevents breakdown of body tissues.

Vitamin K is needed for blood to properly clot, and for the liver to make blood clotting factors, including factor II (prothrombin), factor VII (proconvertin), factor IX (thromboplastin component), and factor X (Stuart factor). Other clotting factors that depend on vitamin K are protein C, protein S, and protein Z. Deficiency of vitamin K or disturbances of liver function (for example, severe liver failure) may lead to deficiencies of clotting factors and excess bleeding.

Amino Acids: The Foundation of Our Body

There are 18 different amino acids, or protein types, that are the building blocks for a healthy body. **Non-essential amino acids** are proteins that the body can synthesize by itself, provided there is enough nitrogen, carbon, hydrogen, and oxygen available. **Essential amino acids** are proteins supplied by the food you eat. They must be consumed in your diet as the human body either cannot make them or cannot make them in sufficient quantities to meet your body's needs.

Proteins act as enzymes, hormones, and antibodies for your immune system. They maintain fluid balance and keep the levels of acid and alkalinity in check. Proteins also transport substances such as oxygen, vitamins, and minerals to target cells throughout the body. Structural proteins, such as collagen and keratin, are responsible for the formation of bones, teeth, hair, and the outer layer of skin and they help maintain the structure of blood vessels and other tissues.

Enzymes are proteins that facilitate chemical reactions without being changed in the process. Hormones or (chemical messengers) are proteins that travel to one or more specific target tissues or organs, and many have important regulatory functions. Insulin, for example, plays a key role in regulating the amount of glucose in the blood.

The human body also uses protein to manufacture **antibodies** (giant protein molecules), which combat invading antigens. Antigens are usually foreign substances such as bacteria and viruses that have entered the body and could potentially be harmful. Immunoproteins, also called immunoglobulins or antibodies, defend your body from possible attack from these invaders by binding to the antigens and inactivating them.

If these critical components for a healthy body are not provided as part of a healthy diet, your body will look for other sources for them. This can include the breakdown of your organs, leading to chronic problems such as liver and kidney problems, diabetes, and heart disease.

Moringa Oleifera Leaf Powder

Moringa is considered a complete food because it contains all of the essential amino acids required for a healthy body.

DRIED MORINGA LEAF is a nutritional powerhouse and contains all of the following amino acids:

ISOLEUCINE builds proteins and enzymes and it provides ingredients used to create other essential biochemical components in the body, some of which promote energy and stimulate the brain to maintain a state of alertness.

LEUCINE works with isoleucine to build proteins and enzymes which enhance the body's energy and alertness.

LYSINE ensures your body absorbs the right amount of calcium. It also helps form collagen used in bone cartilage and connective tissues. In addition, lysine aids in the production of antibodies, hormones, and enzymes. Recent studies have shown lysine improves the balance of nutrients that reduce viral growth.

METHIONINE primarily supplies sulfur to your body. It is known to prevent hair, skin, and nail problems, while lowering cholesterol levels as it increases the liver's production of lecithin. Methionine reduces liver fat and protects the kidneys, which reduces bladder irritation.

PHENYLALAINE produces the chemical needed to transmit signals between nerve cells and the brain. It can help with concentration and alertness, reduce hunger pains, and improve memory and mood.

THREONINE is an important part of collagen, elastin, and enamel proteins. It assists metabolism and helps prevent fat build-up in the liver while boosting the body's digestive and intestinal tracts.

TRYPTOPHAN supports the immune system, alleviates insomnia, and reduces anxiety, depression, and the symptoms of migraine headaches. It also is beneficial in decreasing the risk of artery and heart spasms as it works with lysine to reduce cholesterol levels.

VALINE is important in promoting a sharp mind, coordinated muscles, and a calm mood.

Non-Essential Amino Acids in Moringa

ALANINE is important for energy in muscle tissue, brain, and central nervous system. It strengthens the immune system by producing antibodies. Alanine also helps in the healthy metabolism of sugars and organic acids in the body.

ARGININE causes the release of the growth hormones considered crucial for optimal muscle growth and tissue repair. It also improves immune responses to bacteria, viruses, and tumor cells while promoting the healing of the body's wounds.

ASPARTIC ACID helps rid the body of ammonia created by cellular waste. When the ammonia enters the circulatory system it can act as a highly toxic substance which can damage the central nervous system. Recent studies have also shown that aspartic acid may decrease fatigue and increase endurance.

CYSTINE functions as an antioxidant and is a powerful aid to the body in protecting against radiation and pollution. It can help slow the aging process, deactivate free radicals, and neutralize toxins. It also helps in protein synthesis and presents cellular change. It is necessary for the formation of new skin cells, which aids in the recovery from burns and surgical operations.

GLUTAMIC ACID is food for the brain. It improves mental capacities, helps speed the healing of ulcers, reduces fatigue, and curbs sugar cravings.

GLYCINE promotes the release of oxygen required in the cell-making process. It is also important in the manufacturing of hormones responsible for a strong immune system.

HISTIDINE is used in the treatment of rheumatoid arthritis, allergies, ulcers, and anemia. A lack of histidine may lead to poor hearing.

SERINE is important in storing glucose in the liver and muscles. Its antibodies help strengthen the body's immune

Moringa Over Medicine

system. Plus, it synthesizes fatty acid sheaths around nerve fibers.

PROLINE is extremely important for the proper function of your joints and tendons. It also helps maintain and strengthen heart muscles.

TYROSINE transmits nerve impulses to your brain. It helps overcome depression; improves memory; increases mental alertness; plus promotes the healthy functioning of the thyroid, adrenal, and pituitary glands.

Here are a few of the many nutritional benefits of Moringa Oleifera, the Miracle Tree:

PROTEIN: Moringa leaves are about 40% protein, with all of the 9 essential amino acids present in various amounts (histidine, isoleucine, leucine, lysine, methionine, phenylalanine, threonine, tryptophan, valine). Moringa is considered to have the highest protein

Moringa Over Medicine

ratio of any plant so far studied on earth. Moringa has protein quality and quantity similar to soy beans, but there are no reports of Moringa triggered allergies so it can be used for baby nutrition replacing soy. Moringa is not genetically modified or altered by humans.

VITAMINS: Moringa is a vitamin treasure trove. The amounts of beta-carotene, Vitamin C and Vitamin E found in Moringa exceed those amounts commonly found in most other plants.

Beta-carotene (pro-vitamin A): Moringa leaves contain more beta-carotene than carrots, about three to five times more, ounce per ounce. There is about 7-8 mg of beta-carotene in 100g (about 3 oz.). The daily recommended value is about 1 mg. The body produces Vitamin A from beta-carotene. It is believed that Vitamin A is the most important vitamin for immune protection against all kinds of infections. It is involved in healing and bone development. Beta-carotene guards

Moringa Over Medicine

against heart disease and can keep harmful lipoproteins containing cholesterol from damaging the heart and coronary arteries. It also helps prevent certain types of cancers and stroke. To provide the best anti-cancer protection, beta-carotene should be present with Vitamin C and Vitamin E, and Selenium. Moringa has them all.

Vitamin C: Just one ounce of Moringa leaves contains the daily recommended amount of Vitamin C (60 mg). In fact, it is so rich in Vitamin C that, ounce per ounce, it contains 6 – 7 times that found in orange juice. Vitamin C strengthens our immune system and fights infectious diseases including colds and flu.

Vitamin E: Moringa contains large amounts of Vitamin E, at 113 mg per 100 g (about 3 oz.) of the dried leaf powder. The recommended daily intake of Vitamin E is 10 mg. Vitamin E is a potent anti-oxidant that helps prevent premature aging and degenerative diseases including heart disease, arthritis, diabetes and cancer. It also protects the body from pollution, increases stamina and reduces or prevents hot flashes in menopause. It promotes young-looking skin, as well as healing and reducing scar tissue from forming.

Vitamin B1 (Thiamin): Moringa leaves contain high amounts of Vitamin B1 even compared with the best sources already known. It is higher than green peas, black beans (boiled) and corn (boiled). Vitamin B1 is vital for the production of energy in each cell and it plays an essential role in the metabolism of various carbohydrates.

Vitamin B2 (Riboflavin): Moringa leaves compare with broccoli and spinach in Vitamin B2 content. Vitamin B2 is required for the production of energy, proper use of oxygen and the metabolism of amino acids, fats and carbohydrates. It is needed to activate vitamin B6 and assist the adrenal glands. It is important for red blood cell formation, antibody production and growth. And it is required for healthy mucus membranes, skin, and for the absorption of iron and certain vitamins.

Vitamin B3 (Niacin): Moringa leaves and pods contain about 0.5 – 0.8 mg of Vitamin B3 per 100 grams (about 3 ounces). Recommended daily intake is 18 mg. Vitamin B3 is important for energy production and metabolism of protein, fats and carbohydrates. It supports the function of the digestive system and promotes healthy skin and nerves. Vitamins B1, B2 and B3 work synergistically.

Choline: Moringa leaves and pods contain about 423 mg of Choline per 100 g (3 oz.). Diet recommendations call for about 400-550 mg/day. Choline is critical for normal membrane structure and cellular function. It is used by the kidneys to maintain water balance and by the liver for synthesis of various compounds. It is used to produce the Important neurotransmitter acetylcholine. It is also vital for the developing fetus and infant.

MINERALS:

Calcium: Ounce per ounce, Moringa leaves contain far higher amounts of calcium than most plants, and 4 times the amount of calcium found in milk. Calcium builds strong bones and teeth and helps prevent osteoporosis.

Iron: Ounce per ounce, Moringa leaves contain over three times the amount of iron found in roast beef, and three times that found in spinach. Iron is necessary for many functions in the body including formation of hemoglobin, brain development and function, regulation of body temperature and muscle activity. Iron is essential for binding oxygen to the blood cells. The central function of iron is oxygen transport and cell respiration.

Potassium: Bananas are an excellent source of potassium but ounce per ounce, Moringa leaves contain three times the potassium of bananas. Potassium is essential for the brain and nerves.

Other minerals that Moringa contains include selenium, zinc, magnesium, phosphorus, copper and sulfur.

ESSENTIAL FATTY ACIDS: Moringa Oleifera leaves and seeds contain beneficial essential fatty acids (EFA's). Moringa seeds contain between 30-42% oil, with 13% saturated fats and 82% unsaturated fatty acids. Oleifera is the Latin term for "oil containing." About 73% of the Moringa oil is oleic acid, while in most beneficial plant oils, oleic acid only contributes up to 40%. Olive oil is about 75% oleic acid, and sunflower is about 20%. Oleic acid is linked to lower rates of cardiovascular disease, neurological disease, artherosclerosis, infections, and certain types of cancer, and it helps to regulate blood glucose levels.

OTHER NUTRIENTS FOUND IN MORINGA:

CHLOROPHYLL: Moringa is one of the few foods that contain chlorophyll together with so many other nutrients. Chlorophyll is often referred to as the 'blood of plants." Studies have shown that it supports liver function and detoxification of the body.

BETA-SITOSTEROL: Beta-sitosterol is a specific plant sterol which has been shown to reduce blood cholesterol levels and also improve other blood lipid levels, bringing them to a more normal range. Plant sterols like beta-sitosterol are also proven to be very beneficial in preventing and treating prostate enlargement due to aging, and have been found to reduce the growth of prostate and colon cancer cells. Beta-sitosterol also boosts the immune system, has anti-inflammatory properties,

Moringa Over Medicine

helps normalize blood sugar, supports the pancreas, helps to heal ulcers and can alleviate cramps.

ZEATIN: Biochemical analysis has revealed that the Moringa leaves and leaf powder contain unusually high amounts of plant hormones named cytokinins, such as zeatin and the related dihyrozeatin. Scientists have found zeatin in very low concentrations in plants, with zeatin concentrations varying between .00002 mcg/g material to .02 mcg/g. The zeatin concentration in Moringa leaves gathered from various parts of the world was found to be very high, between 5 mcg and 200 mcg/g material, or thousands of times more concentrated than most plants studied so far.

Cytokinins function as plant hormones, which are naturally occurring growth promoters and factors that delay the process of aging in many plants. In cultured human cells, cytokinins have proven to delay biochemical modifications associated with aging. Zeatin has potent antioxidant properties, and has been shown to protect the skin and increase the activity of known antioxidant enzymes that naturally fight aging. It has also been shown to protect animals against neuronal toxicity induced by age specific factors, and in the laboratory setting, to inhibit cancer cell growth and induce their differentiation back into normal cells.

LUTEIN: Moringa has extraordinary amounts of lutein. 100 g of leaves contain more than 70 mg, while the recommended daily amount for the best protective antioxidant activity is 5 – 20 mg for an adult. Lutein promotes healthy eyes by reducing the risk of macular degeneration.

CAFFEOYLQUINIC ACIDS: Moringa leaves contain 0.5 – 1% caffeoylquinic acids, coming very close to the content that makes artichokes famous. Caffeoylquinic acids are antioxidants considered to be choleretic (bile increasing which helps to digest dietary fats), hepatoprotective (effective against hepatitis and other liver diseases), cholesterol-reducing, and diuretic.

NOTE: Complex mixtures of naturally occurring antioxidants from plants are the most effective and beneficial protectors against oxidation and aging. Moringa contains many other antioxidants including alpha carotene, xanthins, kaempferol, quercetin, and rutin. **(Sandra Toliver)**

This is God's Superfood that's ready, willing and able to meet your health and wellness needs. The most nutritious plant ever discovered and contains no fillers, additives, preservatives, etc… just 100% Superior Grade Moringa Oleifera.

Moringa Over Medicine

"And all the days that Adam lived were nine hundred and thirty years and he died." Genesis 5:5

6

A New You Today, The Moringa Way

"Moringa Oleifera is God's Superfood, it's more than just a vitamin or mineral supplement, it's a way of life."

Your life can change for the better and you've learned a lot in this book but there is much more about Moringa. This is a plant that God has created that is inexhaustible because of the continual unfolding revelation that is been revealed about what it can do for the human body.

When God created mankind from *"the dust of the ground" Genesis 2:7* his body was whole and complete with nothing lacking and nothing missing. For the scripture says, *"And God saw everything that he had made, and, behold, it was very good." Genesis 1:31a*

But after the fall of man his body begins to deteriorate because man had disobeyed God in eating of the forbidden tree. God commanded him saying, *"Of every tree of the garden thou mayest freely eat: But of the tree of the knowledge of good and evil, thou shalt not eat of it: for in the day that thou eatest thereof thou shalt surely die."* Now we know that man did eat of the tree and physically he did not die immediately. However, he did die spiritually immediately for his spirit inwardly became dead towards God and his physical body followed suit many years later.

When God created man he was full of the life of God, he did not have eternal life but he had the breath of God in his being and he was really alive. It took Adam over 900 years to die physically because his physical body was permeating with the life of God and it had to learn how to die through deterioration. *"And all the days that Adam lived were nine hundred and thirty years and he died." Genesis 5:5* The body of Adam begin the process of becoming progressively worse. His health begin to decline, fail, collapse, drop and go on a downward slump until it had no more life in it. His once vibrant body began to descend from a higher level pulsating with life to a lower level of feebleness and eventually death.

Mankind has gone physically from been able to live to a ripe old age of 969 years old (Methuselah) to an age of merely 70 years if he's fortunate enough to live this long. His body has unfortunately deteriorated to the point that at times he/she only lives a few years in the case of children dying with diseases ravaging their bodies.

Mankind in this life will never see the days of 900 years ever again on this side of life, only during the 1000 year reign of Christ and when the new heaven and new earth is established. Nevertheless, we still need to take care of our temple which is our body to the best of our abilities. We need to take better care in the form of dietary, exercise and supplying our body with what it's deficient in on a daily basis.

Daily, you have all kinds of diseases and sicknesses that's pulling on your body and trying to invade your cells and enter your bloodstream to make you sick. Many times your body will fight off these things because God has created it to resist many foreign enemies that shouldn't enter it. However, when your body is deficient in the essential vitamins and minerals that's there to assist you these enemies will have a loophole and enter through an opening that's unprotected and lack resistance.

Many essential vitamins and minerals are there to aid, help and assist our bodies in the fight to protect us but when they're lacking the door is opened. Let's look at some essential vitamins and minerals that help protect and sustain our health and can keep us in tip top shape when they're operating in our body in abundance. Here are the essential vitamins:

1. *Vitamin A*
2. *Vitamin B1*
3. *Vitamin B2*
4. *Vitamin B3*
5. *Vitamin B5*
6. *Vitamin B6*
7. *Vitamin B7 FOLATE*
8. *Vitamin B8*
9. *Vitamin B9*
10. *Vitamin B12*
11. *Vitamin C*
12. *Vitamin D*
13. *Vitamin E*
14. *Vitamin K (K1-Phylloquinone, K2-Menaquinone)*

Moringa Over Medicine

15. Choline
16. Flavonoids

Here are the essential minerals:

1. Calcium
2. Potassium
3. Sodium
4. Magnesium
5. Phosphorus
6. Chloride
7. Trace Minerals
8. Boron
9. Chromium
10. Fluorine
11. Iodine
12. Iron
13. Manganese

Moringa Over Medicine

14. Molybdenum

15. Nickel

16. Selenium

17. Sulfur

18. Cobalt

19. Copper

20. Vanadium

21. Zinc

All vitamins and minerals are necessary for the body to function at optimum but the ones listed above are especially necessary. The beauty of Moringa Oleifera is that all the essential vitamins and minerals are contained within this amazing plant. Since this superfood has come on the scene the day is now over that you will have to go to the store or order online various supplements to make sure that you have your adequate daily supply of vitamins and minerals. No longer will you have to spend hundreds of dollars for various supplements because Moringa has all the nutrients that your body requires in this 1 plant. It's time for a *"New You Today, The Moringa Way."* The product that we have labeled *"God's Superfood"* is ready to enhance your life and take your physical health to a new level of health and wellness.

It's your right as a human being to live your best life and how beneficial is life if you don't have the best of health? It's time to take responsibility for your own health, you only get one body therefore you must do all you can to preserve and sustain it in the best shape possible. It has been wisely stated that *"Your Health is Your Wealth"* for what good is wealth if you don't have the health to enjoy it?

Moringa Oleifera is truly an amazing and remarkable plant that God has created to assist you in your pursuit of good health for good health is God's highest wish for mankind. The word of God states, *"Beloved, I wish above all things that thou mayest prosper and be in health, even as thy soul prospereth." 3 John 2* Right here the word of God shows you that God is interested in the whole man, spirit, soul and body. Not only is he interested but he has given us the remedy to help us fulfill the will of God for our lives in providing Moringa for our physical needs.

Are you ready for a ***"New You Today, The Moringa Way?"*** Then you need to become a partaker and not just a bystander of this amazing product and begin to reap the benefits of a Moringa induced life. The benefits you will derive physically are next to amazing as every organ of your body comes alive as you begin to take life into your body through Moringa Oleifera.

We have seen some truly amazing changes in the lives of individuals that have come into health and wellness through a daily consumption of this remarkable product. Many testimonies of changed lives, sustained lives and lives turned around. You do not have to remain in the state you're in; you can change your life if you're willing to shift to the plant based and whole food supplements of Moringa Oleifera. From taking several different supplements a day to simply taking 1 herb (food) a day, Moringa Oleifera.

In this book we're handing you the physical blueprint to a changed life, this is a book that has the answers you're seeking for physical change. *Are you willing to try? Are you ready to try? Are you ready for a "New You Today, The Moringa Way"?*

7
You Are Fearfully And Wonderfully Made

"I will praise thee; for I am fearfully and wonderfully made: marvellous are thy works; and that my soul knoweth right well." Psalms 139:14

God never originally intended for your body to deal with sickness and disease, it was never a part of God's original plan. God always had high thoughts for mankind and his will is that mankind will be whole in spirit, soul and body. To be whole in spirit yet deficient in soul is still a life out of balance. To be whole in spirit and soul yet deficient in body still isn't God's best for mankind. The word of God says, *"Beloved, I wish above all things that thou mayest prosper and **be in health**, even as thy soul prospereth." 3 John 2*

The will of God for you is total life prosperity. The thoughts of God towards you are precious and he wants your body to be made whole. He says in his word,

Moringa Over Medicine

"My substance was not hid from thee, when I was made in secret, and curiously wrought in the lowest parts of the earth.

16 Thine eyes did see my substance, yet being unperfect; and in thy book all my members were written, which in continuance were fashioned, when as yet there was none of them.

17 How precious also are thy thoughts unto me, O God! how great is the sum of them!

18 If I should count them, they are more in number than the sand: when I awake, I am still with thee." Psalms 139:15-18

God wants your out of balance body to get back in balance because when your body is out of balance it is working against you instead of for you. If your body is currently experiencing any type of disease (dis-ease), illness, sickness, discomfort, ailment, complication, disorder, bug, infirmity, malady, trouble, infection, contagion, attack, bout, fit, feebleness, debility, weakness, frailness, lameness, malady, unsoundness, distemper, epidemic, pest, plague, agitation, disturbance, distress, irritation, etc… then you are not walking in perfect health even though you are fearfully and wonderfully made.

Sickness and disease is not what your body was created for, it's an enemy of your body. Your body was created by your Creator to be healthy and never get sick.

- Sickness is an invasion.
- Sickness is an adversary.
- Sickness is an enemy.
- Sickness is a foreigner.
- Sickness is a negative.
- Sickness is a foe.
- Sickness is an opponent.
- Disease is rivalry.
- Disease is nemesis.

Moringa Over Medicine

- Disease is a curse.
- Disease is an affliction.
- Disease is a minus.
- Disease is a liability.
- Disease is of the devil.

You are fearfully and wonderfully made by your Creator to be full of life with the absent of sickness. However, sickness will not just stay off your body because you want it to, you must do the things necessary not to get sick. Your goal is health and wellness. You want your body to be:

- Full of Life
- Vibrant
- Dynamic
- Healthy
- Flourishing
- Thriving
- Alive
- Robust

Moringa Over Medicine

- Whole
- Fit

From this day forward don't settle for less than the best health. Start to change your ways of eating, your ways of thinking and your ways of living. Begin to make the rest of your life the best of your life.

You were created for purpose and it's hard to fulfill purpose with a sick and diseased body. Take advantage of the privileges that God has bestowed upon you here in America and make your claim to perfect health.

Moringa Oleifera is the one Superfood that stands out above the rest. Right now if you're sick in any form or fashion your body is craving for the 90+ essential nutrients that it needs for satisfaction. Your body wants to get back as close as possible to the feeling of liveliness it felt in the Garden of Eden. It will never get back 100% but it groans to live once again with the feeling of vibrancy.

Moringa Over Medicine

Moringa Oleifera can help equip your body of lifelessness to return to a body of life fullness. I'm telling you this really works, as I'm in my store typing this book today a customer walks in to purchase more products. I take the liberty to ask her how the Moringa Oleifera is working for her. What has she noticed happening in her body? Her response amazed even me; in her own words she stated that:

"It is working great, I've been on Moringa for about 4 months now and I've lost 59 lbs. My aches and pains have left and my energy is back. I can go back to the gym and workout, I feel great." R.B.

She has gotten her life back and she has entered the state of living in her feeling of been fearfully and wonderfully made.

Another testimony of a gentleman that at one point in his life sickness and disease was ravaging his body, he was at a point of great memory lost, he had to give up driving, he was overweight, bloated and walking on a cane. But today his life is different and he's living the good life now. In his own words:

"After using the Moringa Oleifera, my memory begin to return, the bloating left, I was able to drive once again as far as 300-400 miles away without tiredness or memory problem. Today I no longer walk with a cane and I have energy once again." C.B.

He has gotten his life back and he has entered the state of living in his feeling of been fearfully and wonderfully made.

I could go on and on with testimonies one after another of individuals who are now living a better quality of life. A quality that many probably thought they would never be able to live again. It wasn't medicine that gave these individual their life back it was Moringa Oleifera God's Superfood. A revolution is happening and changing people's lives at an astounding rate, don't you want to be a part of it? The Greatest Plant on the Planet is here and it's a life changer. Will you allow it to change your life starting today?

"It's time to live the rest of your life the best of your life and when you supplement with Moringa Oleifera it's like reviving your body daily."

See Our List of Other Books About Moringa:

1. The Greatest Plant on the Planet
2. Moringa Oleifera The Tree of Life
3. The Beelzebub Letters (A serious of 5 books)
4. The Breakthrough Oil That's Changing Lives –Moringa Oleifera

Moringa Over Medicine

**Eden Wellness Moringa
123 N. Center Street
Goldsboro, NC 27530**

www.edenwellnessmoringa.com
edenwellness@yahoo.com

Moringa Over Medicine

Moringa Over Medicine

Moringa Over Medicine

Moringa Over Medicine

Moringa Over Medicine

Moringa Over Medicine

Made in United States
Troutdale, OR
06/16/2024

20538903R00080